Respect Your Hunger Through Intuitive Eating

Listen to Your Body and Conquer Weight Loss Without Diets or Exercise

John Lynch

Copyright © 2020 John Lynch

All rights reserved.

ISBN-13: 979-8-6272-2242-4

© COPYRIGHT 2020 BY **JOHN LYNCH** - ALL RIGHTS RESERVED.

The content contained within this book may not be reproduced, duplicated or transmitted without direct written permission from the author or the publisher.

Under no circumstances will any blame or legal responsibility be held against the publisher, or author, for any damages, reparation, or monetary loss due to the information contained within this book. Either directly or indirectly.

Legal Notice:
This book is copyright protected. This book is only for personal use. You cannot amend, distribute, sell, use, quote or paraphrase any part, or the content within this book, without the consent of the author or publisher.

Disclaimer Notice:
Please note the information contained within this document is for educational and entertainment purposes only. All effort has been executed to present accurate, up to date, and reliable, complete information. No warranties of any kind are declared or implied. Readers acknowledge that the author is not engaging in the rendering of legal, financial, medical or professional advice. The content within this book has been derived from various sources. Please consult a licensed professional before attempting any techniques outlined in this book.

By reading this book, the reader agrees that under no circumstances is the author responsible for any losses, direct or indirect, which are incurred as a result of the use of information contained within this document, including, but not limited to, — errors, omissions, or inaccuracies..

CONTENTS

	Introduction	1
1	The Myth of Diets	3
2	Understanding Why We Eat	11
3	What Is Intuitive Eating?	15
4	Principles of Intuitive Eating - Part 1	19
5	Principles of Intuitive Eating -Part 2	39
6	Getting Started with Intuitive Eating	46
	Conclusion	49

John Lynch

INTRODUCTION

Do you ever wonder what it is with weight loss that has almost the whole world running around to achieve it? For thousands of people around the world, weight loss has become something that is completely unattainable, a far-fetched possibility, yet we continue to try harder than ever to achieve it. The astounding number of diets and exercise programs available are a testament to this fact. People jump from one supposedly promising diet to another in search of ultimate health and long-lasting weight loss. But they never find that.

The common man doesn't know or understand what these so-called beneficial diets do to our bodies. In our race to an admirable physique, we don't realize that we are harming ourselves more than we are gaining from these diets.

Aren't you tired of keeping a check on the number of calories consumed? Aren't you tired of having to rein in your cravings, pass up the cheesecake when in reality you'd like nothing better than to dig your teeth into it? If you are anything like me when I was losing weight—or rather, trying to lose weight through these diets—you have more foods on the forbidden food list than on the allowed food list. From fried cashews to strawberry ice cream, cheesecakes to doughnuts, chicken nuggets to sugary candy, I had a list of nearly every conceivable dream food. But right there was the catch. It was all a list of dream foods that I would never get the chance of tasting again in my life, at least not until I had my weight under control. If I did indulge in any of those in moments of weakened self-control, I would drown in a river of guilt. All because I had one doughnut! How in the world one doughnut could tip the scale was beyond my understanding, but that was the common belief and I went with it. When I began my journey of intuitive eating, all of the guilt and struggles with good and bad foods disappeared and simply vanished into thin air. It was like I had a new life, all thanks to intuition.

Intuition is your inner voice. It helps you get the feel of things when you step into something or do anything. Call it your instinct, your sixth sense, your gut feeling, or anything else you can think of, they all stand to say the same. It's your body, your soul, telling you what you need to do and how.

Though many might argue that intuition isn't that dependable of a judge to completely rely on and that you should use your intellect, I'd say, at least in this case of what to eat and what not to eat, intuition is a good enough judge. Your intuition is the most natural communication your body has with you. This, coupled with your acquired knowledge of nutrition, can help you decide what's best for your body and your health. It is like you simply tune into your own body, and it leads the way to good health and natural weight conditioning. Does this sound impossible and far fetched? Bear with me, and we shall see how you can achieve this seemingly impossible dream all because you listened to yourself!

To begin, we will have to break down the fortress of pre-formed ideas and preconceived notions that diets and the weight-obsessed food police have ingrained in us. Even if you aren't someone who has ever really engaged in the dieting world, there is still the possibility of your subconscious mind taking what it reads and sees in the world around you and saving it as what is ideally allowed or not allowed when it comes to eating. Changing our mentality and approach toward food is the first step. Only when this change is conquered can you step into the world of your intuition and conquer troubling weight loss issues and health problems.

1 THE MYTH OF DIETS

Diets don't work. That is the truth of it. The faster we come to realize and accept this reality, the faster and smoother our transition to real health will be. But breaking down mental walls that have been built up through years of subtle subconscious training will not happen in a day. To start, let's first understand what drives people toward going on diets.

Why People Go on Diets

There are a couple of different reasons why someone might opt to go on a diet. Contrary to popular belief, the reason is not always some elaborate fancy.

Health

Maintaining good health and simply trying to be healthy could be a driving factor behind why many turn to diets as a means to achieve that. Someone might want to control their blood sugar levels, or they might worry over their cholesterol levels, their decreasing stamina, imbalanced blood pressure issues, and so on. All of these reasons can spur a person to take their food intake into consideration and opt to start what they feel is the best-suited diet plan for their individual needs. As long as considerable attention is given to the nutritive value of food and the diet plan itself is deemed as essential and unavoidable for their specific health needs, then, by all means, such a diet can and must be followed. If the problematic area of your health is so dire that a diet plan is the only ultimate solution, then you mustn't back down from taking up appropriate dietary measures. As they say, it is all in the intention.

It is only when the intention is simply to stay fit and healthy and doesn't involve any particular health condition that we might question our adherence to such diets and the need for them. Can good health and fitness be achieved through dieting alone? Aren't there more reasonable and viable methods than simply restricting a bunch of foods that can help us achieve the same result? And what if that result was permanent, not temporary?

Thinness and Weight Loss

We have the image of the picture-perfect model who flaunts his or her abs and envious physique on prime-time TV burned into our minds. For us, there isn't any other ideal to aspire to. From newspapers to billboards, TV commercials to radio announcements, magazines to TV shows, everyone is talking about one dream weight loss program or the other. How can all these dreams and aspirations being pumped into us night and day not have an effect on how we feel about ourselves and how we'd like to see ourselves in the near future? Thus, begins the race to size zero, six-pack abs, and so on. Achieving the body that is 'exactly like my favorite celebrity' is our goal now. To get to this ideal that we have set for ourselves, we scurry around looking for the perfect diet.

My friend Alice has moved from one demanding diet to another, all in the hopes that this one will be the one that'll work. From the myriad of diets that have added to her experience, Alice can assure you that none of them truly work. And this is true for anyone who has gone on a diet. Even if one is able to lose a few pounds over the course of a few weeks, as soon as the diet ends, the pounds come back with a vengeance. All those months of food deprivation come down to nothing, just because you are now back to eating frosted cupcakes and scoops of your favorite cookie dough ice cream. How can one believe that a few months' worth of deprivation would last a lifetime? And continuing those diets for long periods of time and adopting them as your lifestyle isn't going to work either. Not to mention, imagine what such diets can do to your self-esteem and your sense of innate happiness when you are away from things that you truly enjoy. How long do you think your inner peace could last eating only salads or fruit bowls, however fancy they may be?

Types of Diets

To give yourself an idea about the increasing absurdity and farfetchedness of diets prevalent nowadays, let's look at some famous diets followed around the world. Though many of these work and offer temporary weight loss solutions, they are just that—temporary.

Ultra Low Fat Diet

This diet requires that you eat an astoundingly low amount of fat. The diet consists of both low fats and low proteins too, concentrating entirely too much on carbohydrates alone. It is a grain-rich diet including few to no animal-derived products. While it might have its advantages in reducing weight drastically in obese people, it has its many disadvantages too.

A no fat and low protein diet basically removes all animal and dairy products and a range of protein-rich plant products too, like beans or legumes. There is no solid science behind this diet plan. Needless to say, limiting fats limits the options of healthy foods too and offers little to no variety in day-to-day meals.

Fruit Only Diet

This diet is prescribed mostly as a strict form of veganism. But studies have shown that instead of expected weight loss due to restricted forms of high carbs, high fiber, and complete avoidance of proteins and fats, it, in fact, results in weight gain. Fruits have a purer form of carbohydrates in the form of various sugars. This causes the dieter to put on weight.

Also, this kind of diet has been known to be dangerous for diabetics. Proteins, fats, and other micronutrients are essential for our bodies to remain healthy. By depriving ourselves of these important nutrients, we run the risk of attracting several health problems.

Water Diet

This is another popular diet that requires you to restrict yourself to simply water or non-caloric fluids for a limited number of days. Most water diets run from three to seven days. While there have been cases where such extreme dieting measures resulted in weight loss, it is equally true that once the diet is stopped, the dieter begins to gain back the lost pounds at a remarkably quick rate. So, the whole exercise seems futile in the end.

Keto Diet

This is an extremely popular diet plan. It supposedly works on the process of ketogenesis in our bodies. This is the process where our body burns fat for energy and produces ketones as a byproduct. The presence of ketones in the blood is taken as a likely indication of our body undergoing ketosis. It has been widely publicized as an extremely effective weight loss diet program.

This program is supposed to keep you feeling full and satisfied. It has a high amount of fats but is very low in carbs and proteins. The keto diet is also known to bring on mental clarity and healthy skin along with weight loss.

But, what most keto dieters will not tell you is that as soon as they hop off the keto diet, these benefits seem to evaporate. You won't be feeling full any longer as you ease yourself into a normal carbohydrate diet. Also, many keto dieters report weight gain once they are off this diet. Keeping your body in a state of ketosis forever is not an ideal situation. Your body needs glucose. Nature created humans to need glucose and carbs in the right amounts for the effective functioning of muscles and other body functions. Depriving your body of what is rightfully and naturally a normal demand of your body is not healthy in the long run. Therefore, though the keto diet has been proven to be of benefit for a few people in combatting weight gain, it is not an advisable way of styling your eating habits.

Fasting Diet

This is another popular weight loss program that is widely propagated as a lifestyle choice and not a diet plan. But it has been known to become difficult to follow after a period of time. You cannot expect yourself to always remain in a fasting state of whatever intensity just to keep yourself in shape and lose those pounds. There is bound to come a time after long, intensive fasting periods where you are simply too tired to carry on the program. While fasting definitely has its benefits, it is advised to observe it for a limited time only. It should not become a lifestyle change, as some people believe.

Slim Fast Diet

This diet allows you to eat up to six times a day while limiting your calorie intake. You are allowed to consume multiple low-calorie snacks throughout the day (with a maximum of five) and one 500-calorie meal, adding up to the allotted six 'meals' in the day. In reality, what you eat isn't considered meals; rather, they are a replacement of actual meals by store-bought snack bars. These snack bars are in no way satisfying and do not satiate your hunger or keep you full. While this diet might result in weight loss, it is not a good enough gain in the end if you are getting several more health issues in return.

Physiological Disadvantages of Dieting

Unreasonably prolonged dieting can cause several vital changes to occur in your body, and not all of these changes are good. There are many physiological disadvantages to dieting, and we shall look at them one after another.

Slower Metabolism

This is the most common and prevalent disadvantage among all kinds of dieting. Diet plans that especially stress a low carb diet cause your body to experience a famine of sorts with glucose. This can trigger your body to go into starvation mode and begin employing energy-saving techniques. To do this, your body slows its metabolism to slow down energy consumption. This is problematic on so many levels. A slower metabolism means you are losing less energy and burning fewer calories. This results in more fat storage and slower body responses.

Tissue Burn

This is a severe disadvantage of extreme dieting plans. When your body is deprived of readily available energy sources in the form of glucose, your body may resort to breaking down cells to generate energy. The basic diet plans aim for these cells to be fat cells so as to achieve weight loss. But this is not the case every single time. Studies suggest that there is a high chance of your body moving to proteins in your muscles to break down and generate energy. This can cause muscle loss, which is not at all an ideal state to be in. This is actually quite damaging to your body. Muscle tissue burn is a serious disadvantage of dieting. And extreme diet plans or even moderate dieting for really long durations can easily result in this phenomenon.

Decreased Focus and Slower Cognitive Abilities

This is another disadvantage of dieting that becomes apparent in more severe low carb dieters. Reduced concentration and slower cognitive abilities come from a severe drought of carbs. Studies have shown that when carbs were regularly eliminated from a group of dieters' meal plans, their memory and focus deteriorated remarkably. These dieters performed terribly in several tasks that tested their memory and cognition, where they had previously performed well. Therefore, it was concluded that dieting had negative effects on one's abilities to concentrate and apply cognition.

Emotional Disadvantages of Dieting

Dieting also has several emotional impacts on the person dieting. As much as dieting sets off physical and physiological processes, it also lays the foundation for many emotional changes in a person.

Feelings of Guilt

Many people stick to diet restrictions religiously, and there are often many restrictions they must follow. It often happens that these restrictions are on the very things that the dieter loves and enjoys having. If, during the diet, their strict self-control slips, the dieter is immediately plunged into feelings of guilt for having eaten the forbidden.

Remember Alice? She regularly felt guilty for consuming the smallest scoops of her favorite butterscotch ice cream. She had moved from one demanding diet plan to another, and they always left her feeling miserable. She went as far as saying that the simplest action of pushing the grocery cart down an aisle of chocolates had her squirming with guilt. Now, none of the people at the grocery store knew her or her weight issues, and they wouldn't have batted an eye at her buying a pack of chocolates, but she was still left feeling guilty. And it was all because she was straying from her self-imposed dieting limitations.

This isn't just Alice; this is true for many dieters around the world. There are very few dieters around the world who are able to contain this guilty feeling by being insensitive to their own desires and what they are missing out on.

Social Withdrawal

Imagine being invited to a party in the midst of a diet. You can't expect a birthday party to serve diet salads or have no cake. What do you do now? You can't attend and not eat; that'd simply embarrass your host. You can't eat either because that would 'imbalance' your diet schedule and leave you feeling guilty. The only option left, and the one most people would choose, is to stay away from the party. This results in a person withdrawing themselves from social circles and events that involve food. This withdrawal cannot leave you feeling positive about yourself. It is bound to make you feel lonely and alienated, even though the alienation is of your own doing.

Eating Disorders

Eating disorders are a common sight in people who go on diets. Restrictive eating for prolonged periods deteriorates a person's mood and outlook on food. Such people are prone to overeating or binge eating.

People on diets are more at risk for developing eating disorders such as anorexia and bulimia. They often also suffer from depression and have low self-esteem due to weight gain and the above-mentioned feelings of guilt. This, in turn, causes them to eat in a disordered fashion, leading to an eating disorder.

2 UNDERSTANDING WHY WE EAT

It is surprising to realize that we eat for a variety of reasons, and hunger is just one of them. We eat because we are hungry, we eat because we have food lying in front of us, or we eat because a bowl of ice cream seems like a good enough way to tackle a stressful situation. Obviously, not all of these reasons can be healthy. Determining the right reason to eat can be crucial in understanding our eating habits and tailoring them to what is healthy.

The Reasons We Eat

Let's now look at a few different reasons behind why we eat. This will help us take an analytical approach to how we act around food.

Hunger

Hunger, obviously, is the primary reason we think of food. It is the reason we humans began our search for food and developed various ways to acquire it, cook it, and consume it. It is the most basic driving force that keeps our food intake constant. No human is ever 'safe' from hunger. And it is a good thing too. We learn to look for and seek food right from the first day of our lives. Newborns have an innate sense of hunger, and they seek out their nourishment in the form of milk quite naturally without having to train themselves in any way. Right from that earliest age, humans are wired to seek things out that can not only satisfy their hunger but also nourish their bodies.

Food Availability

Another reason we eat is that we have food available. If we have food right in front of our eyes, chances are we will probably pick it up and eat it. Be it little candies or elaborate cupcakes, chips or French fries or a bowl of popcorn, we will eat them all if we find them in front of us. The action is done so unconsciously that we hardly realize that we have picked up a candy or a marshmallow from a tray as we passed by. This is because we almost always have something available to eat. We have simple snack foods lying around that we reach for quite unconsciously.

Avoiding Waste

Many people around the world put a lot of value around food and hate to see it go to waste. To avoid this, many opt to eat leftovers that otherwise would have been thrown out. This does not include those who purposely prepare food in surplus or who otherwise like the dish a lot and would even love to eat it the next day. This, instead, is about those who only eat the food because of the fear of throwing it away. While valuing food is an extremely good habit to cultivate, doing it at the cost of one's own health is not very advisable.

Stress and Boredom

Eating under stress is known as emotional eating, and we shall look at it in-depth in the next section. Eating out of boredom is more commonly seen in children and young adults. This age, especially, demands that you be active and on your toes all the time. When such levels of activity are absent, people resort to food to fill up their time and tackle boredom. This is not at all a healthy habit to cultivate. Munching on food to pass the time and keep yourself busy, in fact, encourages you to be even lazier and more inactive. If you are a food lover, then your food addiction goes a step ahead and food, itself, becomes a reason to bypass work and avoid activity.

Emotional Eating

People turn to food to combat sadness and stress, too. I remember how I began to eat uncontrollably when there was a little stress at my workplace. And just as quickly as I took to food when I was stressed, I stopped my uncontrolled eating when I was stress-free. This goes to show how crucial stress can be in cases of disordered eating.

It is important to control the urge to reach for the box of ice cream or the bag of chips when faced with a problem. Instead, one must learn to identify the real issue that is causing the stress, address it, and work toward solving it. Food only gives you a temporary reprieve. It is like a snooze button that lets you avoid facing your issues for a little while longer. Instead, tackle your problems head-on and avoid turning to food for temporary solace. It does nothing but numb your pain and offer an interesting form of diversion through your taste buds.

It has been found that emotional eating is, in fact, the first step to several eating disorders. Eating uncontrollably in times of stress paves the way for eating that way at all times. Even if you have learned to stop yourself when the stress passes, there is still a chance that you can fall prey to this unhealthy lure of food. If you were able to succumb to food as an alternative to stress management, then there is always the chance that you may repeat yourself, and it can go a step further and turn into an actual eating disorder. Therefore, it is best to train yourself to fight your issues without resorting to food and stop that first instinctive reach to the refrigerator when problems arise.

Eating at Diet Start and End Points

Another irregular area when it comes to food is the very beginning and end of a diet plan. At the start of a diet, many people treat their favorite foods as though it is the last time they will see them. For however long the duration of the diet, those favorite foods will have no place on the menu. For this reason, many resort to overeating or uncontrolled eating right before they start a diet. It is like saying goodbye to all the foods you cannot have during the diet. And this actually goes to show why and how very wrong it is to follow diets that require you to give up what you love.

Similar behavior is seen when a diet ends. It is like the freedom to eat is at last achieved. People who have been on stringent diets are more prone to this behavior. For them, the end of a diet means that what was long prohibited is now within reach, and this leads to, again, overeating or uncontrolled eating. Most people resort to binge eating their favorite foods at the end of a diet. Binge eating is nothing short of an eating disorder in itself and leads to many other disorders like anorexia and bulimia.

Such uncontrolled eating is wrong on so many levels. Not only does it undermine all the self-controlling efforts that dieting requires, it also advocates against the concept of dieting itself, along with being a precursor to future eating disorders.

What Is the Right Reason to Eat and Why?

Out of all the reasons we have explored, only one reason is the right one. Hunger is the only reason that should make you think of food and make you reach for it. There is no compulsion to eat only a limited number of times throughout the day. Hunger is your body's signal to let you know your body needs nourishment and energy.

In all the other reasons that we have discussed, no real attention is given to what your body needs and whether it even needs the food you are eating. Not paying mind to your own body's requirements leads your body's nutritional balance to go haywire, and this is what causes you to develop several diseases. In later chapters, we shall see how to rely on your hunger to eat in a healthy way and keep diseases at bay.

3 WHAT IS INTUITIVE EATING?

Intuitive eating is simply listening to your own body tell you what it needs and when. Listening to your body is a natural way of staying healthy because you are supplying your body with what it actually needs and at the right moment. But because we have been programmed right from our childhood to stick to certain mealtimes and because we have our own diet experiences that color our thinking, intuitive eating doesn't come as naturally to us as it rightly should. But this can be easily remedied by growing accustomed to listening to our body signals and not relying on what our preconceived ideas otherwise convey.

The Need for Intuitive Eating

One might ask, what is the need to turn to yet another methodology to maintain good health and keep weight gain away? What is essential to understand here is that intuitive eating is nothing new and doesn't bring any outside influences to help with our health needs. It is exactly as the name suggests. It is what our own body intuitively and instinctively would tell us to do if we could only break the walls holding our inner voice locked down. But before we begin our foray into what steps to take to ease into this process, let's understand who intuitive eating is for and who must stay away from it.

Who Is It For?

Intuitive eating is for almost everyone. If you wish to be healthy, then intuitive eating is for you. Whether you have been a part of a diet before or not is not an issue at all. As much as intuitive eating is anti-diet, it is not only about breaking the diet mentality; it is also about helping people realize that their bodies are good enough judges of what they need. So, even if you haven't ever gone on a diet, you could very well apply intuitive eating in your life and see the healthy changes it brings to your body.

Who Should Stay Away?

One could say that although intuitive eating is probably for everyone, it is a little difficult to let your body take control of your food requirements when you are suffering from a health issue. For example, people with thyroid issues and those who take artificial thyroid hormones would not be able to judge their body signals adequately based simply on their hunger cues. Also, diabetics can, again, find it difficult to base their daily meals around eating intuitively. If you have a health issue that requires you to stick to a certain kind of diet, then intuitive eating isn't for you. Otherwise, everyone and anyone can make good use of this lifestyle change and benefit from it.

Be a Toddler Again

One of the best things about being a toddler is the way a toddler manages their food. At this young age, we are totally under the influence of our inner voice. Our body directs us to eat when we are hungry and stop when we are feeling full. The innate sense of when to eat, when to stop, along with what to eat, is ripe by the age of three years old. This is when parents bring their own pressures, schedules, and time tables that force our bodies to eat allotted portions of food at allotted times only. Before our bodies have this understanding of the three meals a day concept, we function solely on our intuitions. From the age of infants to toddlers, we are adept at recognizing the signals our body gives us with regards to food.

This is why we often see toddlers denying food when they aren't hungry and similarly demanding food when they do feel hungry even if it isn't the 'right' time for a meal, according to us. This innocent intuition that is the driving force of energetic toddlers is squashed by us well-meaning parents when we introduce them to mealtimes and acceptable and unacceptable foods. Our intuition not just guides us to eat at the right times, but it also helps us make the right choice of food. With the help of our intuition, we will be able to choose the food that makes our body feel 'right.' This is the primary reason why intuitive eating is like a rebirth of the toddler age. You go back to being a toddler through trusting your well-being with your own body.

Let's take a moment to pause here and reflect for a while. Why do you think nature gave you that instinct, that intuition, in the first place? Science proves that right from birth, a baby is able to adjust their feeding to how much their body needs. This is true up till the age of three. This built-in sense of understanding your own body's needs couldn't have been in vain, could it? Why is there even a need to change how and when we eat or what and how much we eat? If trusting our instincts was good enough in that age, then it must be good enough in our adult age too, especially when we are a lot more knowledgeable and mature than when we were toddlers. So why does the same instinct not qualify now to help us decide better when it comes to food? Does it not seem baffling to think that we allowed little innocent children who had no prior knowledge about nutrition to be led around by the signals of their bodies while we are hesitant to let those same signals guide us when we are more knowing and informed?

That very same intuition is entirely qualified and extremely reliable in any and every age. And this is exactly what intuitive eating teaches you. Like I said earlier, intuitive eating is nothing new. It is simply pulling out our long-buried food intuition. It is unearthing our real hunger cues and other body signals to help us navigate the food world better. Trusting our body is, in the end, the most natural and correct thing to do.

Now that we have understood what intuitive eating means in reality, in the next chapter, let's go a step further and dig a little more into what is required of us to take the plunge. Remember, intuitive eating needs you to start fresh with a clean slate with no pre-formed ideas coloring your thoughts.

4 PRINCIPLES OF INTUITIVE EATING - PART 1

There are 10 basic principles of intuitive eating. They are like the most fundamental requirements you will have to meet in order to practice intuitive eating to satisfaction. These aren't some undoable difficult rules that will make your life harder; in fact, these are here to make your food journey as smooth and enjoyable as it can be.

Think of these as your steps to climb as you scale the intuitive eating mountain, except that it isn't a mountain at all, it is an experience. Knock off one principle after another in your list as you move higher. Remember, these principles are the key to having the best use of your own intuition. One might ask, why are these rules or principles even necessary? Would it not be sufficient if you simply ask us to eat whatever we like and whenever we want?

But it isn't so simple. It has taken years for us to build those ideas and rules around food that we now live by. Breakfast at 8 o'clock, lunch at 1 o'clock, dinner at 7. More often than not, this is what we stick to. Adding to that is the fake concept of health and what foods are healthy and what aren't. Do you think all these preconceived ideas and concepts can be broken down and brushed away by a mere word from a medical practitioner? If something has taken so long to build, it will at least take a little while, if not equally as long, to bring it down from the roots. This is where the principles come in. Let's now see these principles one by one.

Principle 1 - Reject the Diet Mentality

This is the first step to intuitive eating and the most important of all. Unless and until you have mastered this one principle and applied it thoroughly in your day-to-day life, you will not be able to proceed further and make use of intuitive eating as you should.

What is required of you is that you let go of all that diets have taught you. This includes vague and incorrect concepts of health such as propagating that carbs are bad, sugars are to be avoided, fats need to be burned, and so on and so forth. These need to be flushed out of our minds and our systems. People, nowadays, increasingly believe that being thin is the equivalent to being healthy. This couldn't be farther from the truth. Thinness is no indication of health. There are scores of people around the world who are thin and yet are troubled by a myriad of health issues. Similarly, there are not-so-thin people, too, who are perfectly fine, healthy, and happy. Washing our minds of these misdirecting ideas about health is the goal of the day.

For those who have been on diets and have experienced the roller coaster rides that they are, it is even more important to get out of the diet loop. You have been going from one diet to another, restricting one kind of food or another at all given times. What this does to your mind is to teach it that there is no right way of eating food until there is restriction involved. If you are not denying yourself anything, then you are not quite doing it right. This is a huge problem if you are thinking of adopting the intuitive eating methodology. You need to trust the way you feel when eating something to decide if it is good for you or not. How does it make you feel? Do you like it? Does your body like it? How does your body feel? Answering these questions can be crucial in making the right food decisions.

For example, consider this. You have always liked taking milk or cream with your coffee or perhaps you wish to try it. But the many different diets that you have participated in over the years have taught you that milk or cream in coffee is bad. Taking it plain and black is the best, and it is what is good for your health and your weight. Be it low fat diets, low carb diets, or fasting diets, all would require you to shun the pitcher of milk and cream entirely for the duration of the diet plan. Now, even after a few months of stopping all kinds of diets and eating restrictions, you are still skeptical when you spot a pot of cream. The first thing you need to do here is to rid your mind of the fact that milk or cream is bad for you. Work on this one concept for as long as you need until you truly believe that there is nothing wrong with either of them. Then, you drink your coffee however you like it and let your body decide. What does it tell you when you drink it plain? What does it tell you when you drink it with milk or cream? How does it make you feel? Was your body better satisfied with a mug full of plain black coffee or with just a half a mug of creamed coffee?

If you are able to answer those questions satisfactorily, then you have achieved your goal. You need simply to follow what cues your body gives you when you eat or drink something. Take similar steps with any rule that you find yourself unconsciously adhering to. Work as long as you need to break the rule in your mind and then let your body be a judge as you experience the food you were working for. If, while following the concepts of intuitive eating, you feel as though you are back to dieting again, then you are simply not doing it right.

The biggest attraction to diet plans is that they offer weight loss as the main result of their efforts. If you see yourself embarking on the intuitive eating journey with weight loss in mind, then that isn't intuitive eating at all. Although intuitive eating can bring you weight loss, at the same time, it can cause others to gain weight too. It all comes down to what your body feels comfortable eating. Your body decides what suits it and what doesn't, what is good for it and what isn't. In the end, if your intuition leads you away from weight gaining foods, as it recognizes its own needs and priorities, then that is when you might lose weight. But if your body feels happy with non-diet food, then you might gain a little weight, but that does not translate to being unhealthy.

Intuitive eating is anti-diet in the strictest sense. You are in no way restricted from eating what and when you like. This is why intuitive eating is guilt-free. If you sense a feeling of guilt creeping up on you while you eat a particular food, a slice of cheesecake perhaps, then that isn't intuitive eating and you are required to break down the walls of guilt marring your experience. As we discussed earlier, guilt is the byproduct of diets, and the presence of guilt shows that somewhere there still exists a piece of diet mentality in our minds, and we need to work on it. Along with guilt comes the knowledge of the supposed 'rule' that we were breaking in the first place that led us to feel guilty. Work on that to remove it from your system entirely so that the mere sight of another slice of cheesecake does not bring the same hesitation in you.

Principle 2 - Respect Your Hunger

This is the second most important principle to internalize as we move ahead on our intuitive eating journey. Learning to identify your hunger and respecting it with an answer offering of food is crucial to intuitive eating. Many dieters equate hunger with embarrassment. It is like a part of you that you wish to hide and not acknowledge. Feeling hungry and satisfying it with food is seen as a sign of weakness among many dieters. If you are dieting, it is as though you are automatically supposed to suppress the feelings of hunger.

There are a few pointers that need to be kept in mind with respect to hunger. What is it biologically? What drives it? And what happens during it?

Digestive Readiness

At the time your body is expecting food, it readies itself with several little changes that occur in your digestive system that help your body prepare itself in anticipation of food. Your brain directs your digestive tract to get ready for the coming of food by releasing different chemicals in your body that trigger the 'hunger' signals.

Saliva

There is a marked increase in the levels of saliva your salivary glands produce at times of hunger. Mouthwatering is the first reaction to hunger by our bodies even when there are no real mouthwatering dishes in sight. This might not be too discernable for some, yet the secretion of saliva is a gift at times of hunger. Saliva is necessary to make the passage of food easier in the digestive tract. It also has important digestive enzymes of its own such as amylase. This increased salivation is a sign that your body is expecting food. This is also why a simple sight of a scrumptiously fried chicken leg, reading an interesting article on cake decorations, or even a casual mention of an apple pie in a discussion triggers a similar salivary reaction in our bodies. Our brain is in anticipation of the foods being discussed or read about. This is not necessarily hunger, but it helps us understand how our body reacts to the expectation of food.

Digestive Hormones

A similar reaction occurs in the rest of the digestive system where increased digestive hormone secretions occur. This is true for everyone experiencing hunger and can be easily manifested in dieters too, both before and after they have eaten, further proving the fact that what they eat is not honoring the needs of their bodies in the right sense.

The NPY Signal

This is a chemical called the Neuropeptide Y. This is released by the brain when it feels the need for carbohydrates in our body. This is when we feel hungry to eat carbs of some kind. Carbohydrates are essential to our body to fuel any and every function that occurs within the cells. For every bodily function, our body requires the readily available energy source or, in other words, glucose. When the glucose stores expire in our bodies, it turns to the next ready source, the glycogens. These are another form of carbohydrate derivatives. When these glycogen stores are also used up by our body, our body turns to the next most readily available source. Now, this could be proteins or fats. Diets run on the belief that it is the fats that are used. But this is not entirely true. Because, even if your body does burn fats in the ketosis process, this produces ketones, which are not usable by almost half of the neuronal cells in the brain. They need either carbohydrate-generated energy or, if that isn't available, they use proteins.

Imagine it like this. You have a fire burning in your fireplace. If you run out of wood, what do you do? Do you pull apart your wooden beams and pillars in the house to feed your fire? Or do you bring in fresh wood to feed it? Carbs and proteins are no different. When you run out of carbs, you mustn't pull proteins out of your muscles to meet your energy needs. It is carbs your body needs, so it is carbs you should feed it. Letting your body take muscle protein might serve the purpose or meet the energy demands, but it will weaken your muscles, and you lose muscle strength and structure, just as you would lose the structure, strength, and beauty of your home.

This is what NPY is trying to tell you. With elevated levels of NPY in your blood, your brain is trying to convey that what you need is carbs. Dieters pointedly ignore the NPY signals during their diets. This has drastic effects on the muscle integrity in the body, as we just saw. This is hunger for carbs and must be satiated by carbs alone. Diets that specify low carb meals deprive your bodies of carbs at an astounding rate. This causes NPY levels to shoot to an abnormal level by the time the next meal arrives, and this is what makes controlled eating even more difficult. It isn't you losing control of yourself; it is your body telling you biologically that you need more glucose. This is another factor that proves that there is no reason to feel guilty at all. It isn't you who is overeating. In fact, what you can feel guilty of is depriving your body of the much-needed carbs in the first place!

Denying Hunger

Dieters are often guilty of this crime. They are more often than not plagued by troubling questions such as, do I deserve this much food? Have I earned it? Has my body earned it? Is the portion too large? This leads them to deny hunger when it knocks on their door. Imagine yourself as you wake for the day. Your body has already experienced a night-long fast. It is literally screaming for energy, for food. If your diet doesn't include fasting by skipping breakfast, then you might eat something, thankfully. Yet, if you are anything like a normal dieter, there are chances that you find your breakfast too large and your body undeserving of so much food so early in the day. What do you do? You skip your lunch. By the time dinner arrives, your hunger is in overdrive and you are nothing less than ravenous. This causes you to overeat, completely undermining the very 'sensible reasoning' that led you to skip lunch in the first place. The vicious cycle continues and you repeat the same pattern day after day, mindlessly forcing your body to undergo strenuous chemical changes just because you are not mindful enough of what you are eating.

Denying hunger results in two kinds of reactions in your body. In one reaction, you eventually overeat after you have initially driven thoughts of hunger from your mind by controlling yourself without giving in to your hunger. In the second and more serious of the two, you lose the ability to listen to your hunger. You are not able to hear your body telling you it needs food. By continuously avoiding responding to hunger signals, you lead them to eventually fade away from your system. When you begin ignoring your body's hunger cues, your body tries even harder to get your attention by sending stronger signals. But when you ignore those too, these signals become inconsequential after a time and you become unable to recognize them. Only extremely ravenous hunger will now be able to get your attention since anything light and subtle has lost its appeal entirely.

A rule of thumb to follow, though not very strictly, is to not go more than six hours without food. This is because it takes around five to six hours for the glycogen reserves in your liver to be used up, and by the end of six hours, your body will need more carbs and more food. It is important to understand that your hunger doesn't just help you eat food that makes you feel full, but it actually is a way for your body to tell you it needs to catch up on energy. This is another reason why diet food is not so good for your body.

Dieters, in particular, resort to foods that keep you feeling full for longer without really giving you any true energy. People drink diet sodas, black coffees, or eat bowls of salads to counter the hunger pangs. They fail to realize that hunger is not just your body's need to fill your stomach; it is also a call for energy. And you need actual carbs to do so. If you eat a couple of diet meals to keep hunger at bay, your body's energy needs aren't met, and it will send even stronger cues the next time because it intends to catch up on the energy reserve too.

Types of Hunger

Hunger that can cause you to reach for food can be one of two types. And there is nothing wrong with satisfying either of them.

True Biological Hunger

This is when your body is in actual need of energy and gives you the appropriate signals. This kind of hunger must always be answered with what you feel like eating and how your body feels as you eat them. These are true biological chemical changes occurring in your body and must not be ignored or left unanswered.

The Hunger of Five Senses

This is when you feel 'hungry' or compelled to try a dish just because you like the way it looks, it smells, it tastes, or it feels. You might listen to the name of a dish and find yourself intrigued and feel like trying it out. This isn't hunger in the true sense, but this is your body's natural response to food too. There is absolutely no harm in indulging your body in satisfying these food desires. True hunger cannot be the only reason for you to have food. Imagine yourself at a friend's house. You are not particularly hungry because you have just had your lunch. But the chicken smells heavenly and the cake looks delish. Would you be wrong in indulging your senses a little by having either of those? Absolutely not. As long as your actions are in response to cues from your body, then they are legitimate and can be followed.

Principle 3 - Food Isn't Your Enemy

What we saw in the previous principle was your body's biological response to the absence of food. This absence could be due to a fast, a dieting plan, or simple time gaps between normal day-to-day meals. But what we are about to discuss, in this principle, is how the absence of food affects you psychologically. It is the long-known truth of basic human psychology that what is out of our reach and denied to us has the most lure in our minds. Let's understand this concept with food.

Imagine a starving little child who's probably not eaten a decent meal for months. If you give him a plate with three slices of pizza and ask him to eat just one and then leave the room, what do you expect to find when you return? Obviously and naturally, the child would have eaten all the three slices of pizza. This is because he was so deprived of that food for such a long time that his brain screamed to make the most of it when it was available.

There are two things to glean from this example. One, if the pizza slices or any food in this particular example were as easily available to the little child, it wouldn't have held such an attraction. The child would have felt secure knowing that food is available in case he feels like having any. Second, depriving someone of something makes us crave it even more. The fact that the child hadn't had a slice of pizza for so long was enough for him to devour it when he found it. This brings us to the most important aspect that people struggle with when it comes to food—cravings.

Cravings and Diets

Cravings are irresistible desires for a particular kind of food. The concept behind cravings is a common enough phenomenon for humans. Humans have seen and experienced a variety of cravings in the form of pregnancy cravings, cravings due to stress, or cravings from a lack of sugars in the body. But another entirely different kind of craving is when a dieter experiences it. Dieters are regularly supposed to forego one or another kind of food for the sake of their diets. Be that ice cream, chocolates, cheese, or whole carbs in the form of bread or potatoes, it is widely seen that the dieter develops an unsatisfiable craving for the very food that is forbidden to them.

My friend Alice was once on a diet that completely removed every trace of chocolate from her diet. Now, Alice was a self-professed chocoholic. She absolutely loved it. These diets were making her miserable, denying her the one and only thing she couldn't live without (her sentiment!). When she did get in touch with a bar of chocolate, she devoured it like she had been starving for years, and then she spent days feeling guilty about it. It was like she was berating herself for befriending the wrong person! Chocolate, the thing she most loved, had now become an enemy of sorts. It was now the one thing that was going to destroy her dieting effort and throw off her weight. Naturally, she kept oscillating between extreme love for the thing and a heightened aversion for it at the same time.

Once she began her journey with intuitive eating and she made peace with the supposed enemy, Alice was at peace herself. She had to realize that chocolate wasn't her enemy for tipping the scales. As she began to give herself free rein over the amount of chocolate she could eat, she was surprised to know how little she actually ate. All this time when she avoided chocolate and then ate it uncontrollably, she was scared to actually let herself be free around it. Rather, she discovered that it was her intense craving for it that led her to eat it at such a fast rate because it was denied to her. Once she made peace with it, though, she did not feel the intense cravings as before. The cravings faded with the freedom she gave herself. She was able to stop herself with a bite or two! Isn't that refreshing and liberating to imagine?

You won't need to fear your eating getting out of control when you are in the vicinity of your forbidden foods. If you can help your mind understand and accept that eating something is not that big of a deal and one or two helpings is not going to tip the scales either way, you will be surprised to see how much less you eat without any effort. This is not some roundabout way of dieting instead. Your mind is actually at ease around those foods. So much so that those cravings will subside to give place to a simple bite or two that will actually be satisfying for you. You may, by all means, take more of the food if your intuition tells you to, but it has been widely seen that once the thing that is so craved is brought within reach, it loses its charm and isn't that attractive anymore. So even though you will still eat it and enjoy it, only a little will be enough to satisfy your inner urges.

Deprivation Scenarios That Trigger Overeating

It is not surprising to see that dieting alone is not the only way one can be deprived of a particular kind of food. There are various scenarios that cause a sense of deprivation in us or, at the very least, trigger a fear of being deprived that, in turn, results in overeating at the first opportunity.

Competition and Fear

Imagine your favorite brand of tomato sauce is stopping

production and, instead, is introducing an entirely different kind of sauce in its place. What do you do when you go grocery shopping? You load your cart with almost every available bottle of the sauce you can lay your hands on. It is like you are in competition with the other buyers and want all the favorite sauce bottles for yourself for fear of being deprived. You fear the time you won't be able to taste it again, and that spurs you to load up the cart.

Or imagine yourself sitting before the television set with a cousin watching a show with a bowl of caramelized popcorn between you. You notice the cousin is a fast eater and is fast finishing the bowl. How do you react? You stuff your mouth with as much popcorn as you can because, again, you fear you'll be deprived of the snack if you do not act now. This is how a sense of competition and fear can push you to overeat and overindulge in something that otherwise wouldn't have gained such a reaction from you.

Away from Normalcy

If someone is away from home for however long a duration due to work or some other reason, then that person is naturally away from the regular food that they are used to eating. This timed deprivation can trigger an overeating reaction when that person comes back home.

Imagine if you or your child is out camping in the woods. Naturally, they are not able to eat the regular foods that they would otherwise eat daily. So, when they come back to the 'normalcy' that they were deprived of, this can urge them to binge eat for a while. Thankfully, though, this kind of binge eating lasts for a limited time only. As soon as the person feels that his body has covered up for the missed food, the binge eating is bound to stop.

These situations are not harmful or wrong in the direct sense. Rather, they work to explain how deprivation or even the fear of it can trigger overeating and how really wrong true deprivation can be. This is why intuitive eating is so anti-diet. A diet deprives you of food, making it your enemy, something that is to be avoided and shunned at all costs. Something that wakes up an avalanche of guilt when consumed.

What you need is to make peace between your food choices. Emotionally, choosing between a scoop of ice cream and an apple must be equal to you. That is the level of comfort you must adopt with your food choices. Only then can you be able to make the right choice of food for your body and not feel guilty about it. This can only happen when we erase from our minds the inherent concept that a particular food is good or bad for us. No food is good or bad on its own. It is how it makes you or your body feel individually that matters. What makes you feel wonderful might not interest me at all. What makes me overjoyed may make you feel revolted. This can happen. And it is essential that we acknowledge this huge truth in our journey of intuitive eating.

You are supposed to eat what you want, what your body wants. Irrespective of whether it is believed to be good or bad food, if your body wants you to eat it, no harm can come of it. This needs to be etched into our minds. That is truly the beauty of intuitive eating. It is the elimination of this factor of fear and guilt and making friends with your food choices that actually sets you free in the end. No doubt, this might look too overwhelming, impossible, or even terrifying now. But once you begin to treat all food choices equally emotionally, you will notice a remarkable difference in your approach to food and how truly happy you can be around food without the stress of weight gain, diet controls, guilty pleasures, and deprivation fears.

Principle 4 - Silence the Food Brigade

Years ago, during my struggle with weight gain through various diets, I once stopped at an Indian fast food pop up stall that sold custom made Indian snacks. I ordered a dosa, a kind of savory pancake that's particularly a south Indian delicacy. I made the unforgivable mistake of requesting extra cheese as the topping for it. The lady next to me reprimanded me fiercely for that extra bit of cheese. No wonder then that the dosa lost its charm that day for me.

What that lady did to me that day is a pretty common occurrence for chronic dieters. You find the food police or the food brigade ready to pin you down as guilty for your food choices. These reprimanding voices can be divided into two categories. Your own voice that stops you from making the choice you wish to make, and the voice of the world around you.

The Internal Food Brigade

This is your own voice that prevents you from eating the food of your choice. You wish to eat that bagel, but your inner food police screams at you to put it right back down. "It's too greasy, too fattening!" it says. What do you do? You give in to the inner rebuke and put the much-desired bagel down. Now, why did your voice stop you? Where and how did it learn that the bagel was greasy, fattening, and simply not good enough for you? This is the result of the diet plans in vogue nowadays all around the world. Even if you are someone who hasn't been on a single diet, your inner voice still stops you from eating that bagel. Why could that be? It is because you and your inner voice, as a result, have picked up on things that you read, learn, and hear around you. This feeds into your conscience and works to police you around food as it sees fit. The only way to silence your inner food policing voice is to reject the diet mentality. The very first principle comes into play again here. The more thorough your rejection is, the more effective your control over the food police can be.

The External Food Brigade

This is a combination of various factors and elements present in the world that contribute to the way you feel around food. These factors can act both one at a time or can influence you all together at once. Let's explore what these various influencing factors can be.

People - Friends/Family/Strangers

The lady in the above example of my experience with a cheese dosa is a classic example of this category of the food police. She was an absolute stranger to me, yet she felt no hesitation in admonishing me for a bit of extra cheese. However well-meaning the rebuke might have been, it is true that she had no say at all in what I chose to eat. Yet, she made it her business to try and stop me from consuming the 'harmful extra calories,' not to mention the 'load of cholesterol.' But this is a common phenomenon all over the world where well-meaning people act in a bid to stop you from spoiling your health.

This is truer in the case of close friends and members of the family. Oftentimes, instead of respecting the choices we make in regards to food, these well-intentioned friends and relatives feel no qualms in reminding us how we are harming ourselves. This can affect us in a myriad of ways. We can grow resentful of the person admonishing us. We may take a dislike to the food we otherwise in reality preferred. We might heed their well-meant yet ill advice and abandon the food. We might realize they mean well and look up to them for more of such advice. Do you imagine any one of these consequences to be good and even mildly beneficial to you? None of them are of any value at all. What you need is to listen to what your body tells you about the food you eat. If it isn't good for you, and you are paying close enough attention to your own body, then it should tell you so, and it will.

All these well-meaning friends, sudden nutrition and health experts, and diet control freaks need to be silenced, and emphatically so. Let the people around you know that you are aware of the choices you are making and are confident about the communication you have with your body. Your body is your kingdom. Let no one, however dear, intrude on the conversations you have with your body. Sternly yet respectfully let these people know that you thank them for their concern, but they need not worry because you are totally in control.

Doing this little act once and saying it loud will help you feel empowered. This might seem like a terrifying prospect. But doing so once will set the path up for all future conversations. These very people will begin to realize and respect you for your choices when they see how happy and in your element you shall be with the food you eat.

Media

The media around us in its many forms is a powerful influencing factor and has quite a huge food brigade of its own. The many television commercials, shows, celebrity interviews, newspaper articles, health and fitness magazines, and so on play an enormous role in how we perceive the food we eat. Constant publicizing of the diet mentality and how thin is good is leaving its mark on our minds. From advertisements and write-ups that celebrate the goodness of diet food and the attractiveness of weight loss programs, our minds are only able to glean just one message: A diet is good and being thin in the goal. These popularizations by the media act as food police on their own. The next commercial on the TV for fiber-rich, cholesterol-free cereal acts as the police for our own choice of cereal. We begin comparing our food choices to what is bandied and shown about in the media.

Adding to this is the pressure of the now prevalent social media channels. All the social media outlets run high trends of the latest fashion diet and how a certain celebrity got to their current size through this or that secret diet plan. Everyone runs around in the race to reach that goal. Unknown to themselves, they are setting up policing factors at every point of their lives. Social media, with its wide open and free atmosphere, becomes a breeding ground for the food brigade. Here, almost anybody is able to comment and condemn anyone. Imagine the effect your single insensitive comment on someone's photograph about their shape or body can have on them!

I recently came across a beautiful ballet dancer who would be termed overweight by the normal weight watchers. She is an excellent dancer and highly talented. Yet most of the comments her dancing pictures and videos received were regarding her weight. Imagine how that must have left her feeling? It was a good thing then that she was a strong woman who took her admonishers head-on.

There is a growing need to silence this kind of food and weight policing. And you can only head down the path of intuitive eating when you are successfully able to shut out the many voices that ask you to reconsider your choice of food and the state of your body.

Nutritional Knowledge

We have been led astray for too long about what kind of food is good for our bodies and what kind is bad. Our accumulated knowledge about the nutritional value of foods and the effects these food items have on our body has been polluted with false information being introduced into the nutrition system. This has left our nutritional knowledge extremely convoluted. What happens as a result is that this misinformation works against our betterment by acting as a passive food police. There is always the fear of crossing the allowed number of calories, consuming more fat units, increasing carb consumption, and so on. We constantly live on the edge of this knowledge trying our best to fall within the nutritional limits we have set for ourselves.

This misinformation is what wrongly informs us that chocolate is bad, carbs need to be reduced, and fats must be eliminated from our diets if we wish to remain healthy. Even those who have never dieted are affected by whatever prevalent knowledge is available about the nutritional value of various foods and our own nutritional requirements of the day.

This is nothing but another form of food restriction that stems from wrong knowledge, however widespread it may be. Therefore, to counter this kind of policing, what we require is to unlearn all the concepts we have about food and relearn the actual facts in the light of intuitive eating. We begin by acknowledging that all food is good. Anything that is remotely diet-like must be eliminated completely. Only then can we truly contain and silence the food brigade within and around us.

Principle 5 - Experience Your Satiety

Just like one needs to identify, acknowledge, and respect their hunger by eating food, one needs to recognize, acknowledge, and honor their satiety or fullness by stopping the eating. This stands true for not just dieters but also all normal non-dieters around the world who are taught right from childhood to finish the food on their plates, to not let food go to waste, to eat till the last guest at the table eats, and so on. There are even weirder rules out there in many cultures that influence a person psychologically to eat past their fullness. There are scores of people who do not know what comfortably full even feels like.

Many would tell you in a moment what uncomfortably full feels like. They feel their food is up to their throats, they can't imagine getting even water in at this point, their stomach feels tight like it's going to burst and so on. But, not one of these people would be able to tell you what just full or satisfied would feel like. Obviously, each and everyone's food experience is different and so is satiety. But, even at their own individualistic level, they would not be able to tell you what it would be like to stop eating when they are simply no longer hungry.

This is because they have never done so. A large number of dieters are included in this group. This is because whatever diet meals they eat are so meager that they never truly experience any fullness, and whatever proper meal they do eat is eaten when they are so hungry that they eat past their fullness cues.

Hormones and Satiety

Our body produces an extremely useful hormone, Leptin, which is otherwise called the satiety hormone. This is the hormone that lets you know when to stop eating. When your body's intake levels have reached a certain level, your body produces Leptin to signal you to stop. In chronic dieters due to deprivation, imbalanced hormones, and starvation for long times, the effects of Leptin are minimal. It is not that they do not still produce this chemical. Rather, their bodies do not quite recognize the signals anymore unless and until they are too full to burst.

Normal, comfortable satiety is exactly that—comfortable. You are content with what you have had and your stomach begins to feel adequately full compared to when you began. Your hunger no longer exists at this point. You can still eat a few more bites, but then that would make you too full. This is the point you need to stop. Stop at the point when you are happy and satisfied with what you have been having and how much you have had.

A golden rule to live by is to never eat large amounts of something that you liked just because you liked it. The chicken was good, but if two or three pieces make you feel good, then stop right there. Just because you are enjoying the chicken, do not ignore the signs of your body trying to tell you it is happy with the amount you have had. Listen to Leptin. The more sensitive you are to this hormone, the better your satiety levels will be. And this need not be so terrifying and ominous. Do not be afraid to listen to your body. And this can be learned and practiced with simple steps too.

How to Recognize Your Satiety

The first step toward recognizing your satiety is to take a self-assessing pause while you eat. As you sit at the table to have your meal, make it a habit, at least initially, to stop at the meal midpoint. Ask yourself these questions as you take your self-assessment break. How do I like the food? Do I like the taste of it? Is my body enjoying the food? Is my hunger still present? How much more do I think I can eat? Have I begun to feel a fullness in my stomach? How does my stomach feel? Is my body saying anything?

These simple yet vital questions can be the key to understanding how your body answers to fullness and satiety. How you are responding to leptin levels in the blood might be entirely different from how someone else might respond. Each individual is different, and their experience of fullness is varied. You need to identify how your body feels when you are full. These questions or something similar along these lines that you feel your body might better be able to answer will help you pin down your own individual fullness experience.

Repeat the process, the self-assessment and the questions, at the next meal. See if you reach a similar state of fullness as you did earlier. A journal will come in quite handy at this point. You can include your fullness experience of each meal, the time it took to arrive at it, the portion of food you ate, your body's responses to the food, and so on. By comparing the various written down notes, you will be able to conclude at what moment you are comfortably full. Remember, the key is to stop at a time when you can still comfortably eat a couple more bites. Beyond that point will begin the overeating arc, and you do not want your body to experience and record overfullness.

Once you have done this exercise a few times, you will be able to experience food in a much more appreciative way as you eat it day after day. You will begin to notice that you enjoy food a lot more, which ultimately adds to your fullness experience. After a few days, you won't need any assessments, charts, or journals; instead, your body will be tuned to stop at the right moment of fullness when you are truly happy and content with what you have eaten.

Factors Influencing Satiety

Now that we have practiced mindfulness while eating and are wiser about the way our body signals fullness, there are a few factors to keep in mind that can, in the end, influence the levels of your satiety.

Time Gap

The time gap between your meals can significantly affect how and when you feel full. If the time gap is less than six hours, you are bound to reach your satiety levels a lot quicker because your body still has reserves of energy from the past meal and, therefore, it signals you to stop sooner.

Type of Food

This also plays an important role in how quickly you experience fullness. If your meal consists of high amounts of protein or fiber, then you will feel fuller sooner. Instead, if your meal comprises more carbs or fats, then you will need more of those in quantity to reach the same level of fullness.

Prior Meals

If you snacked on a chocolate bar or a nutrient bar before you sat for your meal, you are bound to eat less food. What and how much food still sits in your stomach from previous meals or snacks also determines how much you will eat at the current meal and how quickly you will reach your satiety.

Hunger and Company

If you were famished as you sat down to eat, you're naturally going to eat more regardless of your previous meal or the time gap between two meals. This could be because your previous meal was light and got digested sooner though there was no real difference in the time gap. Another reason could be you were involved in some strenuous physical activity that burned your calories quicker, and hence the starving hunger. Whatever the reason for the hunger, the level of it will determine how much you will eat and at what point you will feel full.

Adding to this is the presence of company while you are eating. If you are eating alone, you are more prone to eat less when compared to eating with company. The type of company also affects your food intake. If it's people you enjoy and are comfortable being around, then you will eat more compared to if the company was tiresome or boring; the meal would last a long, boring time, yet you will end up eating less.

At the end of the day, your fullness is yours to experience. Do not let social pressures, workload, or other factors ruin the way you enjoy and experience your food.

5 PRINCIPLES OF INTUITIVE EATING - PART 2

Let's now look at the next bunch of principles that will guide us on the intuitive eating pathway.

Principle 6 - Experiencing the Joy of Eating

In our busy day-to-day lives, eating has become a chore. If not for the attention it gets through diets and health plans, eating would have been a mere part of our background. Even then, the attention it gets makes it not something to enjoy but something to be wary of, something to monitor and tackle, as though it's the monster under the bed. How many times have you eaten a meal and truly enjoyed it? Have you given your taste buds free rein to feel every flavor bursting in your mouth, smell the aromas wafting from the kitchen? Have you given your body the culinary pleasure it craves?

If you can but stop a moment and smell your food, you would be making your body that much happier. A happier body is a happier you. In intuitive eating, making the whole eating process a pleasurable one is important. If you eat with consciousness, relishing every taste and smell emanating from your food, you will be fuller and satisfied for a longer duration. It is like saying that if you are full now, you will eat less later. This has nothing to do with the quantity of food. Rather it is the experience of eating that keeps you happy and feeling fuller. Sounds impossible? Try the following steps to give yourself an enjoyable eating experience.

Steps to Make Eating Enjoyable

Make it a point to give attention to the following details while eating a meal.

Atmosphere or Setting

Sit somewhere that is comfortable and inviting. Pay attention to your own comfort, placement of dishes, having water handy, the comfort of your company, and so on. Do not have meals standing or in areas of the house that are not very convenient.

Taste of the Meal

Pay attention to how the food tastes in your mouth. What taste buds does it stimulate? How do you feel or react to each kind of taste? What other tastes would you rather explore eating?

Texture of the Food

Notice the texture of the food and observe your own reactions to it. Do you like how it feels in your hands? Do you like how it feels in your mouth? Is it hard, soft, rough, grainy, smooth, crispy? What texture do you most enjoy? What other foods might have the same texture?

Smells of the Food

The aromas from the food are as much an attraction as the taste of the food. Do you like the way the food smells? Is there anything you would prefer? What other smells might you enjoy?

How the Food Looks

My dad once said that for a food to be attractive to an eater, it has to pass the appeal test in three different areas. It has to look good, smell good, and finally, taste good. Appearance is the first thing a person notices. Do you like how presentable the food is? Is there anything you would do differently? Do you notice if appearance adds to the appeal of the food?

Hot or Cold

Analyze if you prefer your food hot, warm, room temperature, or cold. What kind of temperature would be best for each kind of food, according to you? I once had a roommate who always had his soup ice-cold, while all the others, including me, would have it piping hot. It appeared weird to us then, but his only constant defense was he liked it that way. Now that I am a practitioner of intuitive eating myself, I can better appreciate his preference for a cold soup even if I still like mine served hot. So look for what works best for you and your body's eating experience.

Quality and Quantity

There might be certain foods that are great to look at, that smell heavenly, and even taste good, but they are not very fulfilling. This might be because the material or quality of food is not meant to be filling, or the quantity is too little. Either way, notice and work around what gives you the best eating experience and make it a point to include only those things that leave you feeling satisfied in the end.

Principle 7 - Handling Emotions Without Eating

Like we have discussed earlier, emotional eating is a precursor to many eating disorders. Turning to food while you are stressed out only pushes you to overeat without any rhyme or reason. One important aspect of intuitive eating is to not let food become a means of fighting emotional wars with oneself. But how does one go about recognizing emotional eating and avoiding it?

Identify Emotional Eating

Emotional eating could be because of a myriad of emotions that a human is capable of. We eat when we are happy and wish to celebrate. We eat when we are stressed, anxious, worried, sad, frustrated, or angry. Oftentimes, emotional eating is not accompanied by true biological hunger and stands on its own. Though this means you are eating beyond your biological hunger cues, it also means that identifying it will be easier because you won't confuse it with any true hunger.

If you find yourself reaching for unusual foods at unusual times, ask yourself the following questions. Am I truly hungry? What am I feeling? Am I tired, sad, angry, or something else? How is food going to help me?

These are difficult questions to answer. And if you really are under an emotional duress, finding yourself in a weakened food-dependent state might trigger an entirely different storm of emotions. It is important, in such situations, to look for help. Would you feel better talking to someone like a friend, family member, or a neighbor? Would it ease your mind and heart if you are able to vent, rage, or simply share your feelings? If no one is available right at that moment, you may simply record your own voice on your mobile phone and play your feelings to yourself. This often gives us a different perspective on how things are.

Remember, your aim here is to solve and confront your issues without the help of food. So take every measure that you think will help you cope with your problems without food. If doing some distracting chore, visiting a friend, doing an interesting activity, listening to music, etc., can help, then, by all means, use those to calm your feelings and keep food out of the equation.

Principle 8 - Loving Your Body

Loving your body just the way it is will be the best gift you can give yourself. The whole dieting system thrives on making us feel resentful and guilty of the kind of body we own. It is as though every other person has the right to ridicule and comment on your body, making you feel ashamed of your own body. We discussed earlier how making peace with food is essential. It is equally essential to make peace with how nature made you.

This isn't to say that one mustn't try to lose weight or that obesity is good. Rather, being in a state of appreciation of your own body gives you a sense of freedom and self-worth that is otherwise lacking in a diet-run system. In their race to lose weight, chronic dieters hardly shed any pounds but lose enormous amounts of self-esteem. And it's all because they feel ashamed of having a large body and affinity for food.

Loving and honoring your body structure and your genes in no way means to undermine the value of health. We need to love our bodies to take better care of them. Exposing our bodies to various diet regimens and what these diets do to us is not taking care of our body. Loving and caring for our body would include feeding it well, taking care of its basic requirements, clothing it as it feels comfortable, and so on. Loving your body also does not necessarily mean loving each and every aspect of your body. Naturally, there might be a few things we do not like. But that, in turn, does not mean we should treat it with harsh diets and strenuous exercises as a means of punishment. This does not feel like love; it feels like retribution for being a plus-size figure.

Principle 9 - Exercise with a Difference

Diets and exercise have often gone hand in hand since they came into being in the weight loss world. You would hardly find a dieter who does not exercise in some way or the other to keep those pounds at bay. Running, jogging, swimming, walking, and lifting weights are just some of the many ways in which dieters opt to burn their calories. If, for some reason, a dieter fails at a diet and stops that particular diet plan, then more often than not, the accompanying exercise also stops because all this time, the enthusiasm of working on a diet was fueling the motivation for the exercise too. The goal here was to lose weight and push along the results to appear sooner. So, automatically, once a diet plan failed and sank, it took with it whatever exercise it was inspiring.

Instead of weight loss, if the goal of doing exercise is to stay healthy, keep active, have better stamina, better confidence, and improved well-being, then it would have been an entirely different matter. In such a case, even if the diet failed, the exercise would have continued. But this is not the scenario we see with most dieters. This is where intuitive eating differs. Once you are at peace with your food choices and your own body, your whole perception of exercise, simple activities, and movement changes dramatically. This is because your goal is not weight loss now.

When you are being an intuitive eater and exercising regularly, just ask yourself the following questions and notice the difference in your attitude. How does exercise make you feel? Are you able to handle stressful situations and anxiety better now? Are you able to sleep more peacefully and greet each morning feeling refreshed? How do you feel about your general well-being? Are you more energized? Do you have increased stamina and feel happy and rejuvenated throughout the day? Do you begin each day with confidence?

I am sure the answers to these questions would have been different had they been asked to a dieter, unless the dieter was a beginner or in the initial euphoric enthusiasm that accompanies a diet in the beginning. A chronic dieter would never answer these questions positively or even with a hint of enthusiasm.

This goes to show how your approach to food and food ethics can have an impact on your individual activities of the day, including exercise. Just make it a point to move about more with a positive outlook for your day. Choose any form of physical exercise that you are comfortable with and note the difference it brings in your attitude every day.

Principle 10 - Respect Good Nutrition

Eating a balanced diet has been the chant of nutritionists for years. But diet regimes have led us to believe that a balanced diet is not necessary at all. In fact, the various diet plans propose different levels for different nutrients. With the advent of diet plans and the onset of the weight loss mania, the concept of variety in food and variety in nutrients has practically gone out the window. We no longer adhere to the nutritional pyramid to determine how much of each nutrient we need. Instead, each diet plan designer is busy chalking up their own methods to achieve ideal health and effective weight loss through what they deem is the perfect nutritive requirement for our bodies.

Intuitive eating couldn't be farther from their misinformed

practices. More than half of these supposedly successful diets do not conform to any scientific proof of nutritional requirements for human bodies. The need of the hour is to reintroduce the carb, the most important energy-giving food, back into our meals.

What many forget or perhaps do not understand is that we do not need a balanced meal on the table every single day. Rather we need a balanced intake of nutrients over a period of time. What we eat consistently and regularly feeds our nutritional average over a period of time. You wouldn't grow deficient by neglecting a particular nutrient in a meal, nor will you tip your scales anyway by including a few more carbs in each meal. What our body accumulates over time and how it reacts to what it is receiving is what matters in the end. And you would be surprised to find how adaptable our bodies naturally are. If you feed your body an overdose of vitamin C through artificial supplements, your body is bound to throw more vitamin C out by way of urine. If you are lacking in potassium levels, your body will automatically begin absorbing more potassium from the future meals. This is just the beauty of nature and our body's adaptability at work. So, one need not worry over an extra bagel or a spoon or two more of the cheesecake. As long as you are paying attention to what your body is telling you and making your food choices accordingly, you and your body are on the way to contentment and happiness with food!

6 GETTING STARTED WITH INTUITIVE EATING

In this brief chapter, let's discuss a few practical measures that you can take to ease your transition into the intuitive eating lifestyle. Naturally, the intuitive eating methodology goes against the grain of what is normally taught and propagated, and beginning on it with confidence can be tough. Use the following pointers to make your journey smoother and more enjoyable.

Intention

Before you begin your foray into this new experience, make your intentions clear to yourself. Use a vision board, a poster, or some other suitable visual stimulation to remind yourself of your intention and goal. Place these around your house where they are easily visible in areas that you frequent. Keep the knowledge and the goal of the first five principles forefront in your mind as you start off. Write shorthand notations of all the things that you feel you will need reminders for. Ditching diets, breaking diet rules, and so on. Keep these rules handy and easy to revise for you. During the beginning of my own journey, I wore these rules as a band around my wrist. It helped me remind myself of my intention to eat intuitively.

Evaluation

From time to time, make it a point to evaluate yourself and your body's responses to food. Take time to pause and observe your feelings and reactions to food. Evaluate your levels of hunger and satiety from time to time. Take notice of the time and the relative levels of hunger and fullness in your body. How much time goes by to reach a point of hunger? How long are you able to feel fullness in your body? These evaluations will help you make informed decisions about your mealtimes. Also evaluate what kind of food leads to what levels of hunger and fullness alternatively. Each individual's evaluation will bring forth different results so work around what works for you.

Keep a Journal

Jot down your day-to-day experiences with intuitive eating. Monitor your health, your fitness and activity levels, your energy levels throughout the day, your feelings on a particular kind of food, and so on. Writing every experience down will help you go back and assess your body's responses to various food-related scenarios. You will be able to gauge your improvement or deterioration as you move further along with intuitive eating.

Have an Intuitive Eating Buddy

Having an interested friend or an ally during your intuitive eating experience will make things easier and smoother for you. Engage a friend or relative to participate in intuitive eating along with you. Compare your observations and reflections on food and food scenarios with those of your friend. This will help you take stock of your own experiences. As you work on breaking diet rules and prebuilt notions on food, you can be a source of inspiration and motivation for each other.

Make Your Own Non-Restrictive Meals

One way to ensure you are rejecting the diet mentality and making peace with food in the truest sense is to cook your own food or make your own meals. Make it a point to include ingredients that you otherwise avoided and stayed away from in the past. This will help break down food prejudices effectively. Making your own meals can become a crucial tool in motivating you to eat non-restrictive food. But, bear in mind, we do not want cooking to become a tiresome chore for you that can instead hinder you from following intuitive eating. Always go by your comfort levels. If you like and enjoy preparing your meals, then do so. If you are someone who has never been even remotely interested in the process of cooking, then, by all means, stay away from the process. The intent here is to make motivational progress as you eat intuitively.

CONCLUSION

Intuitive eating is slowly but surely gaining ground. It is at last beginning to receive the recognition it rightly deserves. Intuitive eating takes you back to your most natural bodily instincts and works with those feelings to arrive at suitable and beneficial food choices.

Intuitive eating is as anti-diet as one can be. Do not let this methodology become yet another hit and miss with dispirited commitment and insufficient follow-through. If done the right way, intuitive eating can give you long-lasting peace with respect to food. You will be a lot happier around food than you ever were.

Intuitive eating is not meant as another weight loss program. You might lose weight as a result of following this method of eating, but that must never be your goal. Instead, look at it this way. Intuitive eating will lead you naturally to achieve the right weight for your body. If you need to put on weight to achieve your normal ideal for your body, then you will do so. Conversely, if you need to lose weight to achieve your ideal for your body, then you will do so. Trust in your body to make the right decision for you.

Recognizing your body's cues is the crux of the intuitive eating process. This cannot be easy and has to be learned gradually. Changes will not happen overnight, but you will be able to notice subtle changes in your body as you progress. Give yourself and your body enough time to get acclimatized to the new approach to eating. With a little patience and commitment, you can reap tremendous benefits from the intuitive eating approach.

www.ingramcontent.com/pod-product-compliance
Lightning Source LLC
Chambersburg PA
CBHW071126030426
42336CB00013BA/2218